HEALTH ASSESSMENT
An illustrated pocket guide

June M. Thompson, R.N., M.S.
Assistant Professor of Nursing
Prairie View College of Nursing
Texas A & M University
Houston, Texas

Arden C. Bowers, R.N., M.S.
Formerly Associate Professor
Department of Nursing
College of Santa Fe
Santa Fe, New Mexico

Third edition
With 88 illustrations

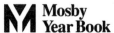

**Mosby
Year Book**

St. Louis Baltimore Boston Chicago London Philadelphia Sydney Toronto

P9-BYG-913

M Mosby
Year Book
Dedicated to Publishing Excellence

Editor: Terry Van Schaik
Developmental Editor: Janet Livingston
Project Manager: Carol Sullivan Wiseman
Production Editor: Diana Lyn Laulainen
Designer: Julie Taugner
Cover Designer: David Zielinski

Third edition
Copyright © 1992 by Mosby-Year Book
A Mosby imprint of Mosby-Year Book, Inc.

Printed in the United States of America.

Mosby-Year Book, Inc.
11830 Westline Industrial Drive
St. Louis, MO 63146

International Standard Book Number 0-8016-6577-9

92 93 94 95 96 GW/PC/PC 9 8 7 6 5 4 3

NOTE TO THE READER

This pocket guide to health assessment is designed as a quick reference for students and practitioners. The outline format simplifies retrieval of material, and the convenient small size makes the guide easy to carry into the clinical area.

The focus of this guide is on the adult client, with considerations for the older adult included where appropriate. General pediatric considerations are also included in this edition. Part 4 presents the examination of the child and developmental guidelines. Part 7 includes growth charts for children.

We have made every attempt to include all the information necessary to make this a complete yet succinct resource for you. We sincerely hope that you will find this guide helpful in your own daily practice.

CONTENTS

PART 1

TOTAL HEALTH DATA BASE

BIOGRAPHICAL DATA

1. Name
2. Age
3. Race
4. Culture
5. Address
6. Marital status
7. Children and family in home
8. Occupation
9. Means of transportation to health care facility, if pertinent
10. Description of home; size and type of community

REASON FOR VISIT

One statement that describes the reason for the patient's visit, or the chief complaint. State in the patient's own words.

PRESENT HEALTH STATUS

1. Summary of patient's current major health concerns
2. If illness is present, include (symptom analysis) history (p. 16)
   a. When was patient last well?
   b. Date of problem onset
   c. Character of complaint
   d. Nature of problem onset
   e. Course of problem
   f. Patient's hunch of precipitating factors
   g. Location of problem
   h. Relation to other body symptoms, body positions, and activity
   i. Patterns of problem
   j. Efforts of patient to treat
   k. Coping ability

CURRENT HEALTH DATA

1. Current medications
   a. Type (prescription, over-the-counter drugs, vitamins, etc.)
   b. Prescribed by whom
   c. Amount per day
   d. Side effects
   e. Problem with compliance

2. **Allergies (describe agent and reactions)**
   a. Drugs
   b. Foods
   c. Contact substances
   d. Environmental factors
3. **Last examinations (note physician/clinic, findings, advice, instructions)**
   a. Physical
   b. Dental
   c. Vision
   d. Hearing
   e. ECG
   f. Chest radiograph
   g. Pap smear (women)
4. **Immunization status (note dates or year of last immunization)**
   a. Tetanus, diphtheria, pertussis
   b. Mumps
   c. Rubella
   d. Polio
   e. Tuberculosis tine test
   f. Influenza

PAST HEALTH STATUS

Although each of the following is asked separately, the examiner must summarize and record the data *chronologically.*

1. **Childhood illnesses**: rubeola, rubella, mumps, pertussis, scarlet fever, chickenpox, strep throat
2. **Serious or chronic illnesses**: scarlet fever, diabetes, kidney problems, hypertension, sickle cell anemia, seizure disorders, blood infections
3. **Serious accidents or injuries**: head injuries, fractures, burns, other trauma
4. **Hospitalizations**: elaborate reason for, location, primary care providers, duration
5. **Operations**: what, where, when, why, by whom
6. **Emotional health**: past problems, help sought, support persons
7. **Obstetrical history**
   a. Complete pregnancies: number, pregnancy course, postpartum course, and condition, weight, and sex of each child
   b. Incomplete pregnancies: duration, termination, circumstances (including abortions and stillbirths)
   c. Summary of complications

FAMILY HISTORY

1. **Alzheimer's disease**
2. **Cancer**
3. **Diabetes**
4. **Heart disease**
5. **Hypertension**
6. **Epilepsy (or seizure disorder)**
7. **Emotional stresses**

8. Mental illness
9. Retardation
10. Alcoholism
11. Endocrine diseases
12. Sickle cell anemia
13. Kidney disease
14. Unusual limitations
15. Other chronic problems

REVIEW OF PHYSIOLOGICAL SYSTEMS

The purpose of this component of the data base is to collect information about the body regions or systems and their function.

1. **General—reflect from patient's previous description of current health status**
   a. Fatigue patterns
      (1) Recent alteration of sleep habits
         (a) Difficulty getting to sleep
         (b) Difficulty staying asleep
         (c) Difficulty getting up in morning
         (d) Excessive napping during day
      (2) Daytime habits
         (a) Unable to stay awake
         (b) Too tired to complete activities of daily living (ADL)
      (3) Describe efforts to regulate sleep
   b. Exercise and exercise tolerance
   c. Weakness episodes
   d. Fever, sweats
   e. Frequent colds, infections, or illnesses
   f. Ability to carry out ADL
2. **Nutritional**
   a. Patient's average, maximum, and minimum weights during past month, 1 year, 5 years
   b. History of weight gains or losses: time element, specific efforts to change weight
   c. Twenty-four-hour diet recall (helpful to mail patient chart to fill in before visit)
   d. Current appetite
   e. Who buys, prepares food?
   f. With whom does patient normally eat?
   g. Is patient able to afford preferred food?
   h. Does patient wear dentures? Is chewing a problem?
   i. Patient's self-evaluation of nutritional status
   j. Is patient on special diet? (describe)
   k. Food consumption pattern
   l. Twenty-four-hour fluid consumption
   m. Chewing problems (describe)
   n. Problem with swallowing (describe)
3. **Integumentary**
   a. Skin
      (1) Skin disease or skin problems or lesions (wounds, sores, ulcers)
      (2) Skin growths, tumors, masses
      (3) Excessive dryness, sweating, odors

(4) Pigmentation changes or discolorations
(5) Pruritis (itching)
(6) Texture changes
(7) Temperature changes
(8) Increased or excessive bruises, excoriation, redness, or trauma marks

b. Hair
(1) Changes in amount, texture, character
(2) Alopecia (loss of hair)
(3) Use of dyes

c. Nails
(1) Changes in appearance, texture
(2) Brittleness, peeling, breaking
(3) Toenails: thickening, difficulty cutting

4. **Head**
a. Headache: characteristics, including frequency, type, location, duration, care for
b. Past significant trauma
c. Vertigo (dizziness)
d. Syncope

5. **Eyes**
a. Discharge (characteristics)
b. History of infections, frequency, treatment
c. Pruritis (itching)
d. Lacrimation (excessive tearing)
e. Pain in eyeball
f. Spots (floaters)
g. Swelling around eyes

h. Cataracts, glaucoma
i. Unusual sensations or twitching
j. Vision changes (generalized or vision field)
k. Use of corrective or prosthetic devices
l. Diplopia (double vision)
m. Blurring
n. Photophobia
o. Difficulty reading
p. Interference with ADL
q. General vision changes
r. Loss of lateral vision
s. Difficulty with night vision
t. Unusual visual effects
u. Difficulty distinguishing colors
v. If bifocals, any problems with adjusting to far vision

6. **Ears**
a. Pain (characteristics)
b. Cerumen (wax)
c. Infection
d. Hearing changes (describe)
e. Use of prosthetic devices
f. Increased sensitivity to environmental noise
g. Vertigo (dizziness)
h. Ringing and cracking
i. Care habits
j. Interference with ADL

    k. Does conversation sound garbled or become distorted?

    l. If hearing aid is used, is it effective?

7. **Nose, nasopharynx, and paranasal sinuses**
   a. Discharge (characteristics)
   b. Epistaxis (nosebleed)
   c. Allergies
   d. Pain over sinuses
   e. Postnasal drip
   f. Sneezing
   g. General olfactory ability
   h. Dry nasal passages/crusting
   i. Painful nose breathing
   j. Mouth breathing

8. **Mouth and throat**
   a. Sore throats (characteristics)
   b. Lesions of tongue or mouth (abscesses, sores, ulcers)
   c. Bleeding gums
   d. Hoarseness
   e. Voice changes
   f. Use of prosthetic devices (dentures, bridges)
   g. Altered taste
   h. Chewing difficulty
   i. Swallowing difficulty
   j. Pattern of dental hygiene
   k. Sore mouth

   l. Dry mouth
   m. Toothache
   n. Loose teeth
   o. Missing teeth
   p. Sores at corners of mouth
   q. Bad breath
   r. Bad taste in mouth
   s. If patient has dentures
      (1) Wearing habits
      (2) Wearing problems
      (3) Cleaning habits and problems

9. **Neck**
   a. Node enlargement
   b. Swellings, masses
   c. Tenderness
   d. Limitation of movement
   e. Stiffness

10. **Breast**
   a. Pain or tenderness
   b. Swelling
   c. Nipple discharge
   d. Changes in nipples
   e. Lumps, dimples
   f. Unusual characteristics
   g. Breast examination: pattern, frequency
   h. Irritated skin under pendulous breasts, rubbing bra

11. **Cardiovascular**
    a. Cardiovascular
       (1) Palpitations
       (2) Heart murmur
       (3) Varicose veins
       (4) History of heart disease
       (5) Hypertension
       (6) Chest pain: character and frequency
       (7) Shortness of breath
       (8) Orthopnea
       (9) Paroxysmal nocturnal dyspnea
    b. Peripheral vascular
       (1) Coldness, numbness
       (2) Discoloration
       (3) Peripheral edema
       (4) Intermittent claudication
       (5) Loss of sensation to pain, touch
       (6) Exaggerated response to cold
       (7) Pain associated with exercise
       (8) Color changes of extremities
       (9) Varicosities
       (10) Does patient wear constrictive clothing?
    c. Heart and hypertension medications: toxicity symptoms

12. **Respiratory**
    a. History of asthma
    b. Other breathing problems: when, precipitating factors
    c. Sputum production
    d. Hemoptysis
    e. Chronic cough (characteristics)
    f. Night sweats
    g. Wheezing or noise with breathing
    h. Painful breathing
    i. Smoking (details)
    j. Exertional capacity
       (1) Shortness of breath with heavy working
       (2) Shortness of breath with exertion at a lower pace
       (3) Shortness of breath with light exertion

13. **Hematolymphatic**
    a. Lymph node swelling
    b. Excessive bleeding or easy bruising
    c. Petechiae, ecchymoses
    d. Anemia
    e. Blood transfusions
    f. Excessive fatigue
    g. Radiation exposure

14. **Gastrointestinal**
    a. Food idiosyncrasies
    b. Change in taste
    c. Dysphagia (inability or difficulty in swallowing)
    d. Indigestion or pain: associated with eating?
    e. Pyrosis (burning sensation in esophagus and stomach with sour eructation)
    f. Ulcer history

g. Nausea/vomiting: time, degree, precipitating or associated factors
h. Hematemesis
i. Jaundice
j. Ascites
k. Bowel habits: diarrhea, constipation
l. Stool characteristics
m. Change in bowel habits
n. Hemorrhoids: pain, bleeding, amount
o. Dyschezia (constipation caused by habitual neglect to respond to stimulus to defecate)
p. Use of digestive or evacuation aids: what, frequency
q. Excessive belching
r. Anorexia
s. Bulimia
t. Bloating
u. Flatulence

15. **Urinary**
   a. Characteristics of urine
   b. History of renal stones
   c. Hesitancy
   d. Urinary frequency (in 24-hour period)
   e. Change in stream of urination
   f. Nocturia (excessive urination at night)
   g. History of urinary tract infection, dysuria (painful urination, urgency, flank pain)
   h. Suprapubic pain
   i. Groin, low back pain
   j. Dribbling or incontinence
   k. Stress incontinence
   l. Polyuria (excessive excretion of urine)
   m. Oliguria (decrease in urinary output)
   n. Pyuria

16. **Genital**
   a. General
      (1) Lesions
      (2) Discharges
      (3) Odors
      (4) Pain, burning, pruritis (itching)
      (5) Venereal disease history
      (6) Satisfaction with sexual activity
      (7) Birth control methods practiced
      (8) Sterility
   b. Men
      (1) Prostate problems
      (2) Penis and scrotum self-examination practices
      (3) Scrotal lumps, masses, or surface changes
      (4) Pain preceding, during, and after erection
   c. Women
      (1) Menstrual history: age of onset, last menstrual period (LMP), duration, amount of flow, problems
      (2) Menopausal history: LMP, any bleeding or spotting since LMP, any related symptoms

(3) Amenorrhea (absence of menses)
(4) Menorrhagia (excessive menstruation)
(5) Dysmenorrhea (painful menses), treatment method
(6) Metrorrhagia (uterine bleeding at times other than during menses)
(7) Dyspareunia (pain with intercourse)
(8) Soreness or pressure sensation in vagina

17. **Musculoskeletal**
   a. Muscles
      (1) Twitching
      (2) Cramping
      (3) Pain
      (4) Weakness
      (5) Manual dexterity problems
      (6) Interference with ADL
   b. Extremities
      (1) Deformity
      (2) Gait or coordination difficulties
      (3) Interference with ADL
      (4) Walking: amount per day
      (5) Problems with shoes
      (6) Restless legs
      (7) Transient paresthesia
   c. Gait
      (1) Any alterations noted by patient: weakness, balance, difficulty with steps
      (2) Walking aids

   d. Bones and joints
      (1) Joint swelling
      (2) Joint pain
      (3) Redness
      (4) Stiffness: time of day related
      (5) Joint deformity
      (6) Noise with joint movement
      (7) Limitations of movement
      (8) Interference with ADL
   e. Back
      (1) History of back injury: characteristics of problems, corrective measures
      (2) Interference with ADL
      (3) Back pain (do symptom analysis)
      (4) Stiffness
      (5) Corrective measures (e.g., use of bed board)

18. **Central nervous system**
   a. History of central nervous system disease
   b. Fainting episodes
   c. Seizure
      (1) Characteristics
      (2) Medications
   d. Cognitive changes
      (1) Inability to remember (recent vs. distant)
      (2) Disorientation
      (3) Phobias
      (4) Hallucinations
      (5) Interference with ADL

e. Motor-gait
    (1) Coordinated movement
    (2) Ataxia, balance problems
    (3) Paralysis (partial vs. complete)
    (4) Tic, tremor, spasm
    (5) Interference with ADL
f. Sensory
    (1) Paresthesia (patterns)
    (2) Tingling sensations
    (3) Other changes
g. Speech
    (1) Unusual speech pattern
    (2) Aphasia
    (3) Dysarthria

19. **Endocrine**
    a. Diagnosis of disease states: thyroid, diabetes
    b. Changes in skin pigmentation or texture
    c. Changes in or abnormal hair distribution
    d. Sudden or unexplained changes in height and weight
    e. Intolerance to heat or cold
    f. Exophthalmos
    g. Goiter
    h. Hormone therapy
    i. Polydipsia (increased thirst)
    j. Polyphagia (increased food intake)
    k. Polyuria (increased urination)
    l. Anorexia (decreased appetite)
    m. Weakness

20. **Allergic and immunological** (Optional; use if patient indicates allergic history. Note precipitating factors in each case.)
    a. Dermatitis (inflammation or irritation of skin)
    b. Eczema
    c. Pruritis (itching)
    d. Urticaria (hives)
    e. Sneezing
    f. Vasomotor rhinitis (inflammation and swelling of mucous membrane of nose; nasal discharge)
    g. Conjunctivitis (inflammation of conjunctiva)
    h. Interference with ADL
    i. Environmental and seasonal correlation
    j. Treatment techniques

21. **Does patient have any other physiological problems or disease states not specifically discussed? If so, explore in detail (e.g., fatigue, insomnia, nervousness).**

PSYCHOSOCIAL HISTORY

1. **General statement of patient's feelings about self**
2. **Feelings of satisfaction or frustration in interpersonal relationships**
    a. Home (occupants)
        (1) If alone
            (a) Is patient lonely?

      (b) Describe access to friends, family
      (c) Does patient feel safe?
    (2) If with family
      (a) Does patient participate in family decisions, activities?
      (b) Does patient have sufficient space, privacy, place for belongings?
      (c) Are there family conflicts? (describe)
  b. Most significant relationship (in and out of home)
  c. Community activities
  d. Work or school relationships

3. Activities of daily living
  a. General description of work, leisure, and rest distribution
  b. Significant hobbies or methods of relaxation
  c. Family demands
  d. Community activities and involvement
  e. During period of day/week is patient able to accomplish all that is desired?

4. General statement about patient's ability to cope with ADL

5. Occupational history
  a. Jobs held in past
  b. Current employer
  c. Educational preparation
  d. Satisfaction with present and past employment
  e. Time spent at work vs. time spent at play

  f. Work/retirement concerns
    (1) Reduced/fixed income
    (2) Role change/loss
    (3) Allocation of time
    (4) Relationship problems with family/spouse

6. Recent changes or stresses in patient's life-style (e.g., divorce, moving, new job, family illness, new baby, financial stresses)

7. Patterns in which patient copes with situations of stress

8. Response to illness
  a. Does the patient cope satisfactorily during own or others' illnesses?
  b. Do the patient's family and friends respond satisfactorily during periods of illness?

9. History of psychiatric care or counseling

10. Feelings of anxiety or nervousness: characteristics and coping mechanisms

11. Feelings of depression: symptoms such as insomnia, crying, fearfulness, marked irritability or anger

12. Changes in personality, behavior, or mood

13. Concerns about aging changes, developmental tasks, sense of accomplishment, and stability

14. Use of medications or other techniques during times of anxiety, stress, or depression

15. Habits
  a. Alcohol
    (1) Kinds: beer, wine, mixed drinks

(2) Frequency per week
(3) Pattern over past 5 years, 1 year
(4) Drinking companions
(5) Alcohol consumption increased when anxious or stressed

b. Smoking
(1) Kind: pipe, cigarette, cigar
(2) Amount per week/day
(3) Pattern over past 5 years, 1 year
(4) Smoking with others
(5) Smoking increased when anxious or stressed
(6) Desire to quit smoking: method, attempts

c. Coffee and tea
(1) Amount per day
(2) Pattern over past 5 years, 1 year
(3) Consumption increased when anxious or stressed
(4) Physiological effects

d. Other
(1) Overeating or sporadic eating (e.g., always in refrigerator, soft drink abuse, cookie jar syndrome)
(2) Nail biting
(3) Street drug usage
(4) Nervous noneating

16. **Physical well-being concerns** (e.g., body image, illness and coping, concerns about dying/death)

17. **Financial status**
   a. Sources
   b. Adequacy
   c. Recent changes in resources and expenditures

HEALTH MAINTENANCE EFFORTS

1. **General statement of patient's own physical fitness**
2. **Exercise**: amount, type, frequency
3. **Dietary regulations**: special efforts (describe in detail)
4. **Mental health**: special efforts such as group therapy, meditation, yoga (describe in detail)
5. **Cultural or religious practices**
6. **Frequency of physical, dental, and vision health assessment**

ENVIRONMENTAL HEALTH

1. **General statement of patient's assessment of environmental safety and comfort**
2. **Hazards of employment**: inhalants, noise, heavy lifting, psychological stress, machinery
3. **Hazards in the home**: concern about fire, stairs to climb, inadequate heat, open gas heaters, inadequate toilet facilities, concern about pest control, inadequate space
4. **Hazards in neighborhood**: noise, water, and air pollution, inadequate police protection, heavy traf-

11

fic on surrounding streets, isolation from neighbors, overcrowding
5. **Community hazards**: unavailability of stores, market, laundry facilities, drugstore, no access to bus
line

SAFETY ASSESSMENT*

1. Gait and balance problems
   a. Slippery or irregular surfaces
   b. Obstruction or clutter
   c. Steep or dark stairs
   d. Bathtub slippery
   e. Shoes without support
   f. Climbing or use of ladder
   g. Clothing too long
   h. Walking in busy traffic areas
2. Decreased vision
   a. Insufficient illumination in home
   b. Glare from polished floor
   c. Missing the bottom step
   d. Bifocals
   e. Medication error
3. Decreased sensation to pain or heat
   a. Hot bath water
   b. Heating pads or hot water bottle
4. Other
   a. Fire hazards
   b. Driving or traffic accidents

*Use this optional assessment if patient is disabled or has difficulty with ADL.

ACTIVITIES OF DAILY LIVING (ADL) ASSESSMENT*

A. Self-care
   1. Dressing, undressing, clothing
      a. Keeping clothes in good repair (mending)
      b. Access to clothes
      c. Getting into and out of underwear (bra, girdle, underpants, pantyhose, stockings, garter belt)
      d. Putting on and removing pants
      e. Getting arms in sleeves
      f. Managing zippers, buttons, snaps (especially in back), ties
      g. Putting on socks, shoes, tying laces
      h. Applying prostheses (e.g., glasses, hearing aids)
   2. Grooming and hygiene
      a. Washing, drying, brushing hair
      b. Brushing teeth
      c. Cleaning and putting in dentures
      d. Shaving
      e. Nail care: feet and hands
      f. Applying makeup
      g. Preparing bath water and testing temperature
      h. Getting into and out of tub, shower

   3. Hearing over telephone
   4. Answering door
   5. Immediate access to neighbors, help
D. Eating
   1. Access to market
   2. Preparing food (opening cans, packages, using stove, reaching dishes, pots, utensils)
   3. Handling knife, fork, spoon: cutting meat
   4. Getting food to mouth
   5. Chewing, swallowing
E. Housekeeping, laundry, house upkeep
   1. Making bed
   2. Sweeping, mopping floors
   3. Dusting
   4. Cleaning dishes
   5. Cleaning tub, bathroom
   6. Picking up clutter (to patient's satisfaction)
   7. Taking out trash, garbage
   8. Use of basement: stairs, cleaning
   9. Laundry facilities: in home or near residence, washtub, clothesline
   10. Yard care: garden, bushes, grass

      i. Reaching and cleaning all body parts
  3. Elimination
    a. Position altered for urination or sitting on
       toilet
    b. Ability to wipe self
    c. Lowering onto and rising from toilet
B. Mobility
  1. Difficulty climbing or descending stairs: is bed-
     room/bathroom on upper level? how many stairs/
     flights to apartment or house?
  2. Sitting up, rising from bed
  3. Lowering to or rising from chair
  4. Walking: short and long distances (describe
     necessity for walking)
  5. Opening doors
  6. Reaching items in cupboards
  7. Necessity for lifting: any difficulty
C. Communication
  1. Dialing telephone
  2. Reading numbers

  11. Other home maintenance concerns (e.g., access
      to fuse box, storm windows, furnace filters,
      painting)
F. Medications
  1. Large number of prescriptions
  2. Difficulty remembering
  3. Ability to see labels/directions
  4. Medications kept in one area
G. Access to community
  1. Bus line
  2. Walking
  3. Driving (self or service from others)
  4. Church, dry cleaning, drugstore, bank, health
     care facility, dentist, other community agencies
H. Other
  1. Caring for spouse/relative/companion
  2. Financial management: able to write checks,
     make payments, cash checks
  3. Care of pet(s)

*Use this optional assessment if patient is disabled.

PART 2 ANALYSIS OF A SYMPTOM

In addition to the health data base, the examiner must be prepared to collect in-depth information about a symptom. The following format is a data collection tool that can be used for physiological, psychological, or sociological symptoms.

CHIEF COMPLAINT

A one-sentence or brief statement using the patient's words to describe the reason for the visit.

ANALYSIS APPROACH

Reconstruction from the patient's words of the body or mental processes underlying the symptom.

1. **Last time patient was entirely well**
   a. Patient may confuse onset of symptom with the first time he was *concerned* about it.
   b. Major symptom may have been preceded by other less alarming ones (e.g., fatigue) that the patient will not recall unless questioned.
2. **Date of current problem onset**
   a. Name specific date and time if possible.
   b. Inquiry about the setting at the time of onset may help establish chronology (time of day, month).
   c. How was patient feeling before symptom onset?
3. **Character** (describe the qualities of the problem)
   a. Move back to quoting the patient (what is the pain like? "like being stabbed"; "squeezed in a vise")
   b. Severity (does it interfere with ADL?)
4. **Nature of problem onset**
   Was the onset slow? Abrupt? Noticeable to others? Use quotes if possible.
5. **Patient's hunch of precipitating factors**
   In determining aggravating or alleviating factors, word questions to avoid influencing answers (e.g., angina: "what effect does walking have?" vertigo: "what happens if you move your head?")
6. **Course of problem** (did patient continue with normal activity during episode?)
   a. Consistent
   b. Intermittent
   c. Duration

7. **Location of problem**
   a. Pinpoint
   b. Generalized, vague
   c. Radiation patterns
8. **Effect on other systems and activities**
   a. Symptoms, signs
   b. Body functions or positions
   c. Activities: body movement, exercise
   d. Eating
9. **Patterns**
   The patient may exhibit a symptom that has been occurring intermittently over a period of time. Most previous questions have elicited data about the quantity and quality of *one* episode. This question concerns multiple episodes, identifies patterns, and provides an overview of chronology.
   a. Timing. Relate incidences to number of times per hour, day, week, month; inquire about patient's well-being during the intervals.
   b. Duration and quality variations. May indicate a stepping up or increase in intensity over a period of time ("has it been getting any better? worse? staying the same?")
   c. If there have been exacerbations or remission, try to associate with other symptoms, activities, or precipitating factors.
10. **Efforts to treat**
    a. Home remedies (what and when)
    b. Body positions (e.g., bed rest)
    c. Over-the-counter medications
    d. Prescription medicines and physician visits (give details)
11. **In-depth exploration of patient's life-style and coping ability as related to the symptom**
    a. Pose questions to discover an association between daily activities and the symptom.
       (1) What mandatory activities make the symptom worse? (e.g., if stair climbing causes chest pain, must patient use stairs at home or at work?)
       (2) What activities are altered or curtailed because of the symptom? (e.g., if the patient complains of nocturnal urination, how much sleep is lost? is fatigue a problem? possible to sleep during the day?)
       (3) Do altered activities pose a threat to the patient? (e.g., if patient complains of diminished vision or glare, is driving hazardous? is reading part of job?)
    b. Pose questions that indicate an association between patient's ability to deal with current life-style and the symptom (e.g., if a mother complains of marked fatigue, does this interfere with childrearing activities or management of the home?)

c. A general question such as "What does this problem *mean* to you?" might help summarize the previous questions. It also permits the patient to voice an emotional response to changes or problems. It may help the examiner grasp more fully the impact or severity of the symptom.

PART 3

PHYSICAL ASSESSMENT GUIDE BY BODY SYSTEMS

GENERAL

1. Temperature
2. All pulse
3. Respirations
   a. Rate
   b. Character
   c. Time inspiratory and expiratory phases for 1 minute
4. Blood pressure (patient sitting and lying)
   a. Right arm
   b. Left arm
5. Height
6. Weight

SKIN, HAIR, AND NAILS

1. Inspection and palpation of the skin
   a. Color, vascularity, and lesions
   b. Symmetry, thickness, and texture
   c. Hydration, turgor, and mobility
   d. Temperature
   e. Hygiene
2. Inspection and palpation of the nails
   a. Color, length, and symmetry
   b. Firmness, texture, and thickness
   c. Adherence to nail bed
   d. Hygiene
3. Inspection and palpation of the hair
   a. Color
   b. Quantity, distribution, and texture
      (1) Pattern of any loss
   c. Condition
      (1) Any infestations
4. Measure nail base angle

Adapted from Moncure F, Miller M, Ball JW, and Dains JE: Instructor's manual to accompany Mosby's guide to physical examination, ed. 2, St. Louis, 1991, Mosby–Year Book.

PRIMARY SKIN LESIONS

Papule

Elevated, palpable, firm, circumscribed, less than 1 cm in diameter, brown, red, pink, tan, or bluish red

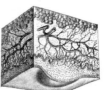

Plaque

Elevated, flat topped, firm, rough (superficial papule greater than 1 cm in diameter, may be coalesced papules)

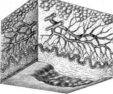

Wheal

Elevated, irregularly shaped area of cutaneous edema, solid, transient, changing, variable diameter, pale pink

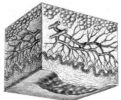

Nodule

Elevated, firm, circumscribed, palpable, deeper in dermis than papule, 1 to 2 cm in diameter

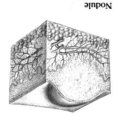

Macule

Flat, nonpalpable, circumscribed, less than 1 cm in diameter, brown, red, purple, white, or tan

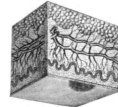

Patch

Flat, nonpalpable, irregularly shaped (macule greater than 1 cm in diameter)

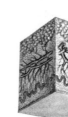

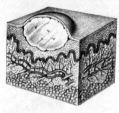

Tumor
Elevated, solid, may or may
not be clearly demarcated,
greater than 2 cm in diameter,
may or may not vary from
skin color

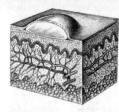

Vesicle
Elevated, circumscribed,
superficial, filled with serous
fluid, less than 1 cm in
diameter

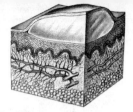

Bulla
Vesicle greater than 1 cm
in diameter

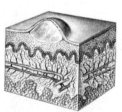

Pustule
Elevated, superficial (similar
to vesicle but filled with
purulent fluid)

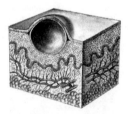

Cyst
Elevated, circumscribed,
palpable, encapsulated, filled
with liquid or semisolid
material

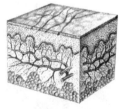

Telangiectasia
Fine, irregular red line pro-
duced by dilation of capillary

21

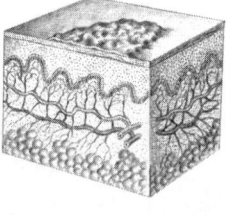

Scale
Heaped-up keratinized cells, flaky exfoliation, irregular, thick or thin, dry or oily, varied size, silver, white, or tan

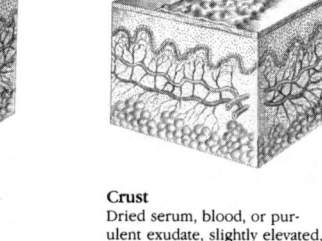

Crust
Dried serum, blood, or purulent exudate, slightly elevated, size varies, brown, red, black, tan, or straw

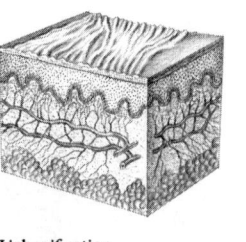

Lichenification
Rough, thickened epidermis, accentuated skin markings from rubbing or irritation, often involves flexor aspect of extremity

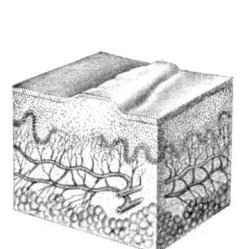

Scar
Thin to thick fibrous tissue replacing injured dermis, irregular, pink, red, or white,

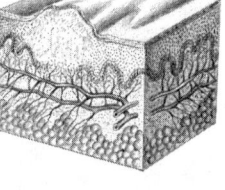

Keloid
Irregularly shaped, elevated, progressively enlarging scar, grows beyond boundaries

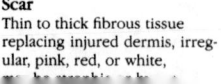

Excoriation
Loss of epidermis, linear or hollowed-out crusted area, dermis exposed

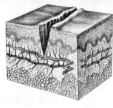

Fissure
Linear crack or break from epidermis to dermis, small, deep, red

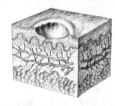

Erosion
Loss of all or part of epidermis, depressed, moist, glistening (follows rupture of vesicle or bulla, larger than fissure)

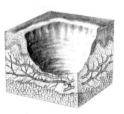

Ulcer
Loss of epidermis and dermis, concave, size varies, exudative, red, or reddish blue

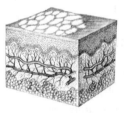

Atrophy
Thinning of skin surface and loss of skin markings, skin translucent and paperlike

23

HEAD AND NECK

1. Inspection and palpation of the head and scalp
   a. Head symmetry, shape, and size
   b. Facial symmetry, shape, and size
   c. Frontal and maxillary sinuses and mastoid process for patency with tenderness
   d. Tenderness, lesions, tics, or unusual features such as deformities, protrusions, or edema
2. Inspection and palpation of the neck
   a. Strength of sternocleidomastoid muscle against resisting hand (can be tested during neurological assessment)
   b. Neck symmetry and range of motion
   c. Trachea position
   d. Thyroid for size, shape, and symmetry
   e. Carotid artery status
3. Auscultation of head and neck areas
   a. Temporal artery for bruits
   b. Over the eyes for bruits
   c. Temporomandibular joint for clicking or crepitus
4. Inspection and palpation of superficial lymph nodes
   a. Size and consistency
   b. Mobility and tenderness
   c. Temperature
   d. Symmetry between sides
5. Inspection of visible nodes
   a. Visibility and position
   b. Edema

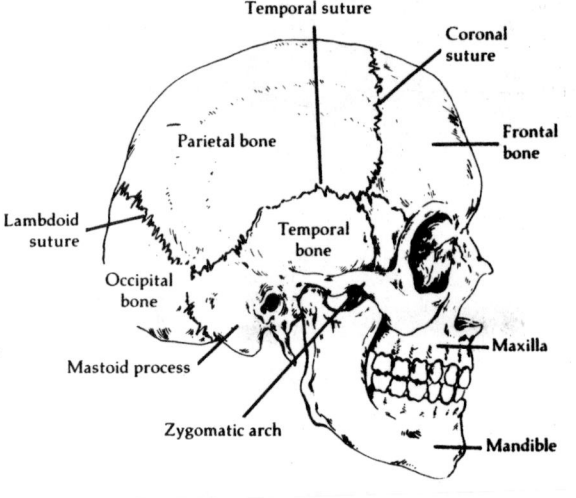

Anatomical landmarks of skull

Temporal suture
Coronal suture
Parietal bone
Frontal bone
Lambdoid suture
Temporal bone
Occipital bone
Mastoid process
Zygomatic arch
Maxilla
Mandible

Anatomical landmarks of lateral head and neck

Anatomical landmarks of anterior neck

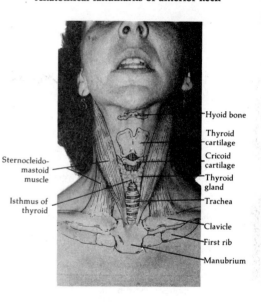

Preauricular

Submaxillary

Submental

Anterior triangle

Postauricular

Occipital

Superficial cervical

Deep cervical

Internal jugular vein

Internal carotid artery

Trapezius muscle

Posterior triangle

Supraclavicular

Clavicle

Sternocleidomastoid muscle (cut and partially removed)

Hyoid bone

Thyroid cartilage

Cricoid cartilage

Thyroid gland

Sternocleidomastoid muscle

Trachea

Isthmus of thyroid

Clavicle

First rib

Manubrium

25

EYES

1. Inspection and palpation of the eyes
   a. Movement of eyes and reaction to light and touch
   b. Pupil condition and response to light
   c. Six cardinal fields of gaze
   d. Lacrimal gland condition
   e. Orbital area
      (1) Any edema, sagging, drainage, or lesions
   f. Eyelids and eyelashes for symmetry, color, quantity, blinking patterns, and distribution
      (1) Any ptosis, tremors, flakiness, lesions, inflammation, or edema
   g. Conjunctivae and sclerae for color and condition
      (1) Any discharge, pterygium, corneal arcus, hemorrhage, or foreign bodies
   h. Corneal clarity (use oblique lighting)
      (1) Any scars, abrasions, ulcers, or cloudiness
   i. Iris for color and condition
      (1) Any bulging
2. Ophthalmoscopic inspection
   a. Lens clarity
   b. Red reflex
   c. Retinal color
   d. Blood vessel characteristics
   e. Disc characteristics
   f. Macula characteristics
3. Vision testing
   a. Visual acuity—near and distant
   b. Visual fields
   c. Corneal reflex

Longitudinal cross section of eye showing focused ophthalmoscope lens settings

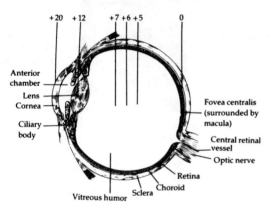

+20 +12 +7 +6 +5 0

Anterior chamber

Lens

Cornea

Ciliary body

Fovea centralis (surrounded by macula)

Central retinal vessel

Optic nerve

Retina

Choroid

Sclera

Vitreous humor

Optic disc landmarks

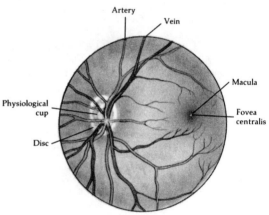

Artery

Vein

Macula

Physiological cup

Fovea centralis

Disc

EARS

1. Inspection, palpation, and testing of the ears
   a. External ear for size, shape, and color
      (1) Helix, antihelix, lobule, tragus concha, moles, cysts, or crystals
   b. External meatus
      (1) Cerumen, discharge, foreign bodies, redness, edema, tenderness, or scaling
   c. Tympanic membrane, cone of light, umbo, handle, and short process of malleus
      (1) Any tenderness, edema, inflammation, drainage, or tinnitus
   d. Weber's test
   e. Rinne test
   f. Whisper or watch test
   g. Romberg test

Ear landmarks

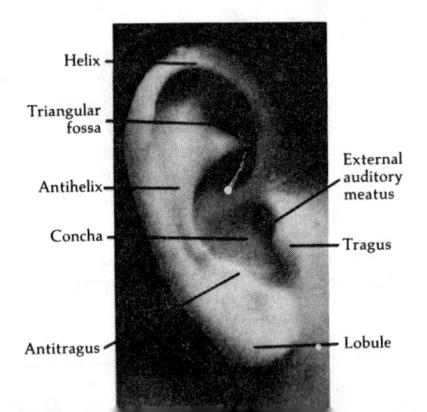

Helix
Triangular fossa
Antihelix
Concha
Antitragus
External auditory meatus
Tragus
Lobule

Tympanic membrane landmarks

Short process of malleus
Manubrium of malleus
Posterior canal
Tympanic membrane
Anulus
Cone of light
Umbo

NOSE AND THROAT

1. Inspection, palpation, and testing of nose
   a. Patency of nares
      (1) Any masses or protrusions
   b. Ability to differentiate odors
   c. External nose for shape, size, and symmetry
      (1) Any lesions, edema, or protrusion
   d. Internal nose color and characteristics
      (1) Any septum deviation, performations, masses, discharges, bleeding, or foreign bodies
   e. Ability to differentiate smells
2. Inspection and palpation of the mouth and throat
   a. Internal and external lips for color and condition
      (1) Any lesions or congenital defects
   b. Teeth and gum characteristics—color, hygiene, mouth odor, number of teeth, spacing, and dental work
      (1) Any plaque, caries, gum bleeding, hyperplasia, inflammation, lesions, or edema
   c. Tongue and frenulum color, size, and condition
      (1) Any restricted protrusion, midline deviation, or twitching
   d. Condition of salivary glands, buccal cavity, and floor of mouth
   e. Uvula and tonsils (if present) for position and condition
      (1) Any exudates, hyperplasia, ulcers, masses, or inflammation

Dentition of deciduous teeth and their sequence of eruption

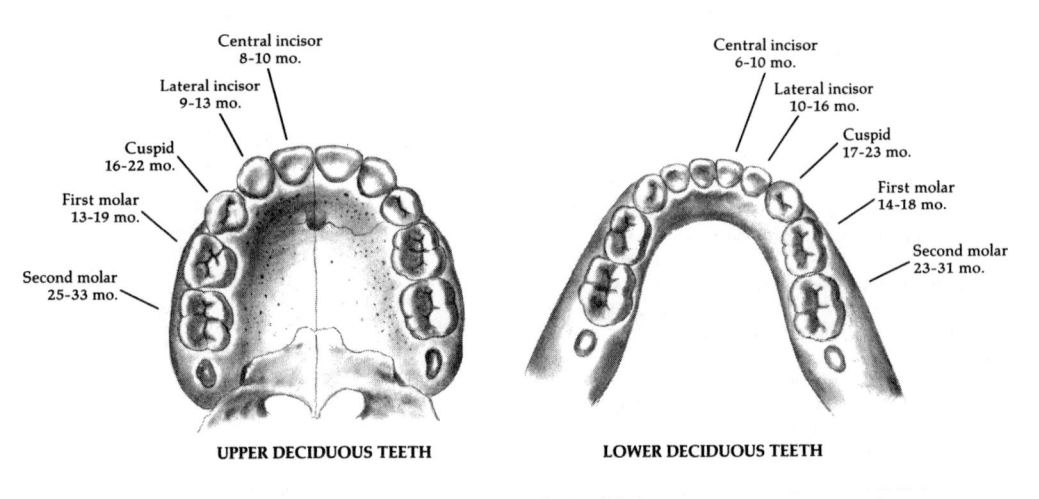

UPPER DECIDUOUS TEETH

- Central incisor 8-10 mo.
- Lateral incisor 9-13 mo.
- Cuspid 16-22 mo.
- First molar 13-19 mo.
- Second molar 25-33 mo.

LOWER DECIDUOUS TEETH

- Central incisor 6-10 mo.
- Lateral incisor 10-16 mo.
- Cuspid 17-23 mo.
- First molar 14-18 mo.
- Second molar 23-31 mo.

Dentition of permanent teeth and their sequence of eruption

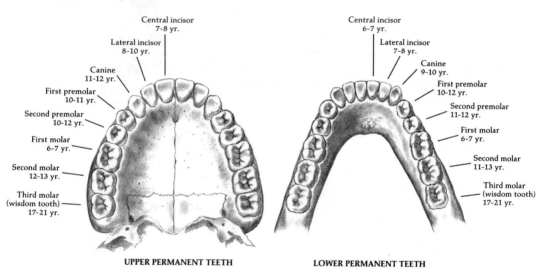

Central incisor
7-8 yr.

Lateral incisor
8-10 yr.

Canine
11-12 yr.

First premolar
10-11 yr.

Second premolar
10-12 yr.

First molar
6-7 yr.

Second molar
12-13 yr.

Third molar
(wisdom tooth)
17-21 yr.

Central incisor
6-7 yr.

Lateral incisor
7-8 yr.

Canine
9-10 yr.

First premolar
10-12 yr.

Second premolar
11-12 yr.

First molar
6-7 yr.

Second molar
11-13 yr.

Third molar
(wisdom tooth)
17-21 yr.

UPPER PERMANENT TEETH

LOWER PERMANENT TEETH

31

CHEST AND LUNGS

1. Inspection and palpation of the chest
   a. Shape, symmetry, and color of front and back
   b. Respiratory rate, rhythm, and effort
      (1) Any retractions, stridor, cyanosis or flaring of nostrils, or pursed lips
   c. Thoracic shape and condition
      (1) Any tenderness, pulsations, bulges, or depressions
   d. Chest wall characteristics
      (1) Any tenderness, masses, or lesions
   e. Chest movements
      (1) Costal or diaphragmatic breathing
2. Percussion, auscultation, and measurement of the chest
   a. Measurement of diaphragmatic excursion
   b. Intensity, pitch, duration, and quality of percussion tones
   c. Rales, rhonchi, wheezes, friction rubs, cough
   d. Lung sounds when patient says "99," "ee," and "one, two, three"
   e. Respirations at rest and 5 minutes after exercise

Topographical landmarks of thorax

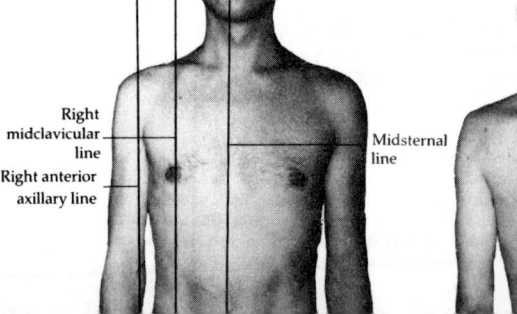
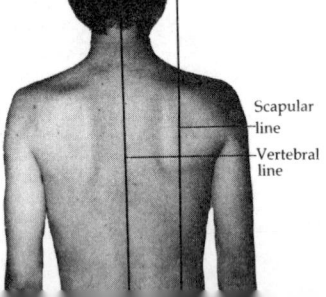
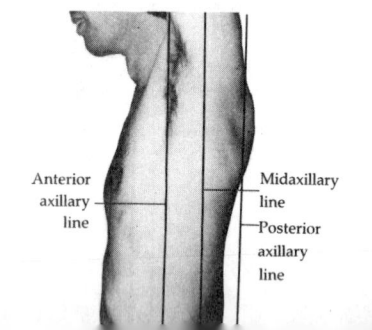

Right midclavicular line
Right anterior axillary line
Midsternal line
Scapular line
Vertebral line
Anterior axillary line
Midaxillary line
Posterior axillary line

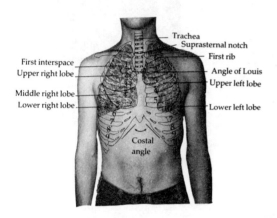

Trachea
Suprasternal notch
First rib
First interspace
Upper right lobe
Angle of Louis
Upper left lobe
Middle right lobe
Lower right lobe
Lower left lobe
Costal angle

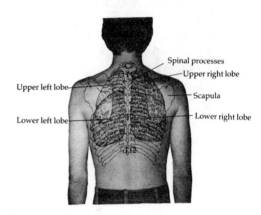

Spinal processes
Upper right lobe
Upper left lobe
Scapula
Lower left lobe
Lower right lobe
T.12

33

Percussion tones of thorax

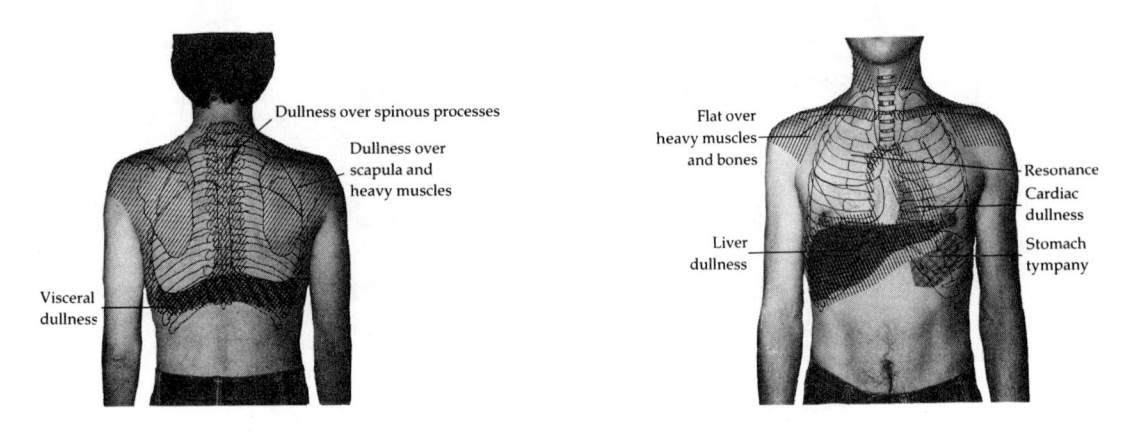

Breath sounds over lung fields

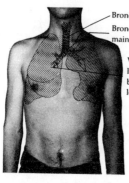

Bronchial over trachea

Bronchovesicular over main bronchus

Vesicular over lesser bronchi, bronchioles, and lobes

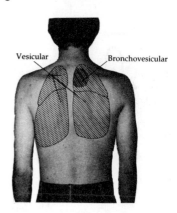

Vesicular

Bronchovesicular

Vesicular breath sounds
Low pitch, soft expirations

Bronchial breath sounds
High pitch, loud expirations

Bronchovesicular breath sounds
Medium pitch, medium expirations

Adventitious breath sounds

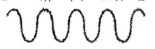

Pleural friction rub: dry, rubbing or grating sound usually due to inflammation of pleural surfaces; heard throughout inspiration and expiration; loudest over lower anterior lateral surface

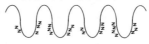

Sonorous rhonchi (wheeze): low, loud, coarse sound like snore; may occur at any point of inspiration or expiration; usually means obstruction of trachea or large bronchi (coughing may clear sound)

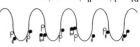

Rhonchi: small airway noise
Sibilant rhonchi (wheeze): musical noise like squeak
May occur during inspiration or expiration, but usually louder during expiration

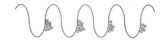

Coarse rales: loud, bubbly noise, heard during inspiration
Found in patients with pneumonia (not cleared by cough)

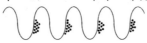

Medium rales: lower, more moist sound, heard about halfway through inspiration
Found in patients with pneumonia or pulmonary edema (not cleared by cough)

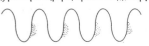

Adventitious sounds, including rales and fine rales, high-pitched crackling sound, heard toward end of inspiration; indicates inflammation or congestion

HEART AND BLOOD VESSELS

1. Inspection and palpation of the heart (patient sitting and supine)
   a. Precordium for pulsation
      (1) Any heave, lift, or thrill
   b. PMI location, diameter, amplitude, and duration
   c. JVP level
2. Inspection, palpation, and auscultation of arteries and veins
   a. Location of palpable pulses
   b. Pulse characteristics
   c. Peripheral veins and capillary refill
      (1) Any insufficiency of varicosities
   d. Allen's test
3. Auscultation of the heart
   a. Rate, rhythm, intensity, and splitting
   b. S1, S2, S3, and S4 sounds
   c. Characteristics of aortic area, pulmonic area, Erb's point, trispid area, and mitral area

Palpation areas for cardiac examination

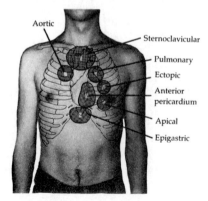

- Aortic
- Sternoclavicular
- Pulmonary
- Ectopic
- Anterior pericardium
- Apical
- Epigastric

Anatomical and auscultatory valve areas

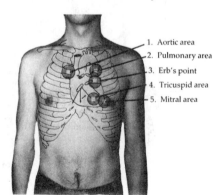

1. Aortic area
2. Pulmonary area
3. Erb's point
4. Tricuspid area
5. Mitral area

**Ventricular systole—
contraction of ventricles**

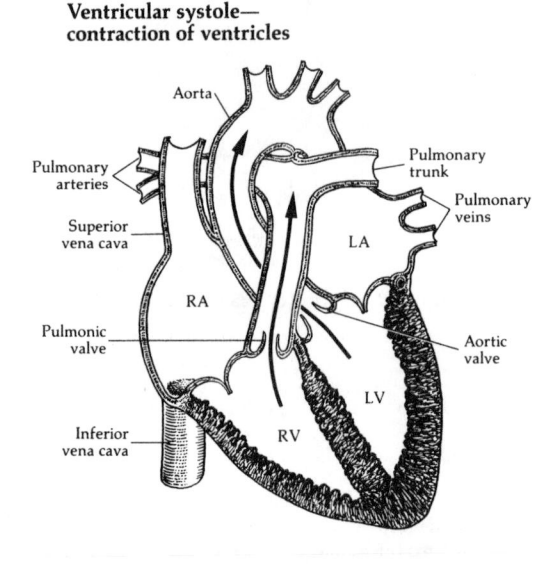

Aorta

Pulmonary
arteries

Superior
vena cava

RA

Pulmonic
valve

Inferior
vena cava

RV

LA

LV

Pulmonary
trunk

Pulmonary
veins

Aortic
valve

**Ventricular diastole—
relaxation of ventricles**

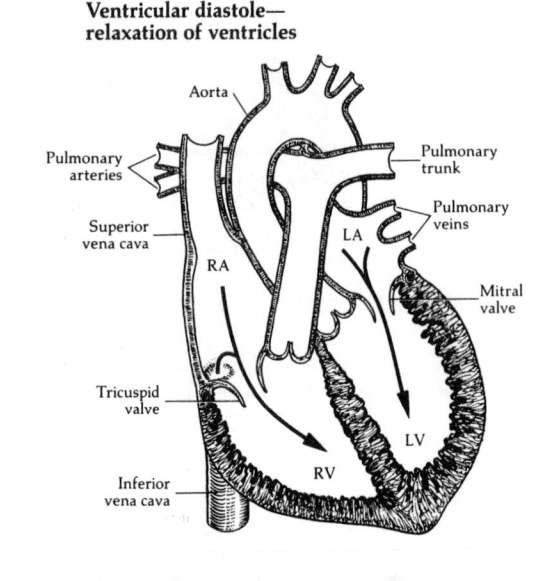

Aorta

Pulmonary
arteries

Superior
vena cava

RA

Tricuspid
valve

Inferior
vena cava

RV

LA

LV

Pulmonary
trunk

Pulmonary
veins

Mitral
valve

BREASTS AND AXILLAE

1. Inspection and palpation of female breasts (patient lying, upright, leaning; range of motion and hand presses)
   a. Size, contour, and symmetry
   b. Color, consistency, and elasticity
      (1) Any tenderness, dimpling, nodules, retractions, protrusions, or supernumerary nipples
   c. Nipple and areolae characteristics
      (1) Any tenderness, inversion, eversion, retractions, discharge, or lesions
2. Inspection and palpation of male breasts
   a. Breast characteristics
   b. Nipple characteristics

Lymphatic drainage of breast

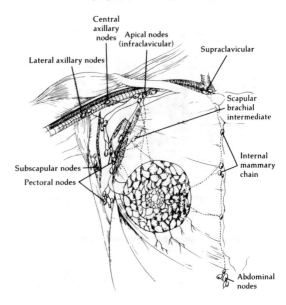

Central axillary nodes

Apical nodes (infraclavicular)

Supraclavicular

Lateral axillary nodes

Scapular brachial intermediate

Internal mammary chain

Subscapular nodes

Pectoral nodes

Abdominal nodes

ABDOMEN

1. Inspection of the abdomen (patient supine, pillow under head, arms at sides)
   a. Skin and umbilical characteristics
      (1) Any inflammation or lesions
   b. Abdominal size, contour, and symmetry
      (1) Any bulges, masses, distention, pulsations, hernia, or peristalsis
2. Auscultation of all quadrants
   a. Bowel sounds and frequency
   b. Liver and spleen areas
   c. Arteries
      (1) Any bruits or hums
   d. Epigastric and umbilical areas
3. Percussion of all quadrants
   a. Tympany
   b. Bladder dullness
   c. Estimation of liver size
   d. Splenic dullness
4. Light palpation of all quadrants
   a. Muscle resistance
      (1) Any tenderness or masses
   b. Inguinal region
      (1) Any bulges or tenderness
5. Deep palpation of all quadrants
   a. Abdominal organs and umbilical ring
      (1) Any kidney tenderness
   b. Aortic pulsation

Major structures of abdominal cavity

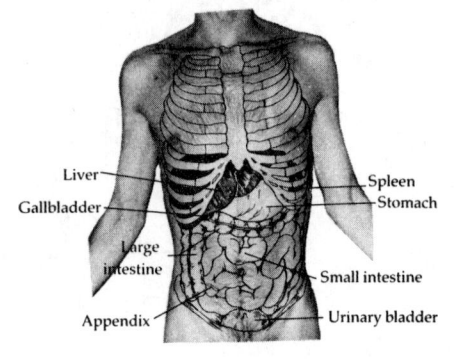

Liver
Gallbladder
Large intestine
Appendix
Spleen
Stomach
Small intestine
Urinary bladder

FEMALE GENITALIA

1. Inspection and palpation of the female genitalia
   (patient in lithotomy position)
   a. Labia and clitoris for symmetry and
      characteristics
   b. Urethral meatus and vaginal opening
      (1) Any discharge or lesions
   c. Perineum for smoothness and muscle control
      (1) Any tenderness, lesions, or inflammation
2. Speculum and bimanual palpation
   a. Cervix characteristics
      (1) Any lesions or discharge
   b. Vaginal characteristics
      (1) Any nodules or masses
   c. Uterus characteristics
   d. Characteristics of ovaries

MALE GENITALIA

1. Inspection and palpation of male genitalia
   a. Penis and urethral characteristics
      (1) Any induration, discharge, or tenderness
   b. Testes and vas deferens
      (1) Any masses or tenderness
   c. Hernia evaluation

Development in females

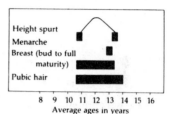

Development in males

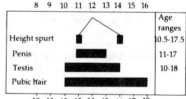

ANUS, RECTUM, AND PROSTATE

1. Inspection and palpation of the anus and rectum
   (Lithotomy, side, and knee chest position)
   a. Sacrococcygeal characteristics
      (1) Any lesions, inflammation, or dimpling
   b. Anal characteristics
      (1) Any hemorrhoids, fissures, lesions, or
          prolapse
   c. Muscular ring and posterior rectal walls
      (1) Any tenderness, masses, or irregularities
   d. Male prostate characteristics

MUSCULOSKELETAL SYSTEM

1. Inspection and palpation of the musculoskeletal
   system
   a. Alignment, contour, and symmetry of bone
      structure
      (1) Any deformity
   b. Muscle characteristics—against resistance
      (1) Any edema, spasms, masses, atrophy, or
          irregularities
   c. Range of motion and function of joints
      (1) Neck
      (2) Shoulder
      (3) Elbow
      (4) Wrist
      (5) Hip
      (6) Knee (drawer test, McMurray's test)
      (7) Ankle and foot

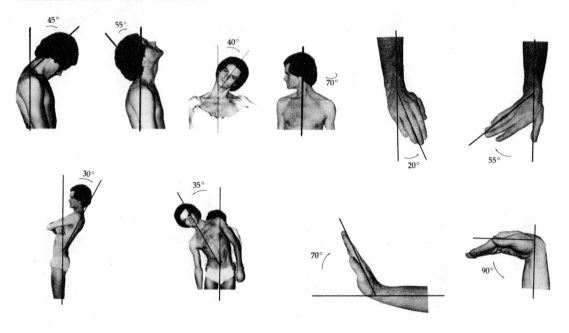

Musculoskeletal functional assessment

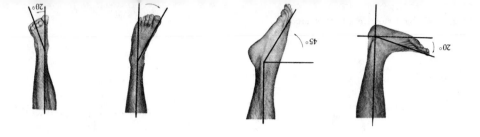

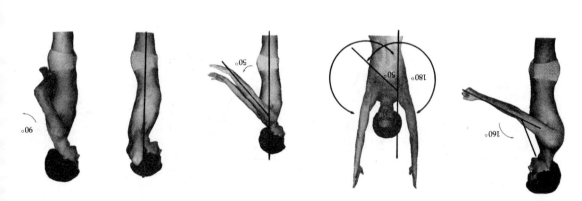

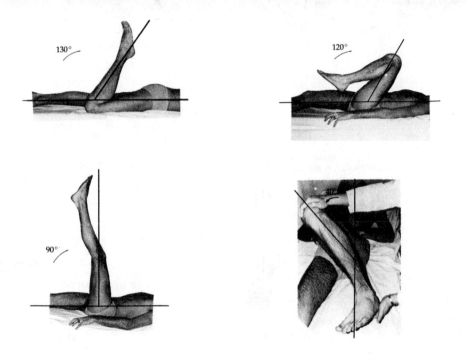

NEUROLOGICAL SYSTEM

1. Inspection, palpation, and neurological tests
   a. Mental status
      (1) Appearance and behavior
   b. Balance, gait, and hand and leg coordination
   c. Reflexes
      (1) Biceps
      (2) Triceps
      (3) Brachioradialis
      (4) Abdominal
      (5) Knee
      (6) Ankle and plantar
   d. Motor function—upper and lower extremities
   e. Sensory function—upper and lower extremities
      (1) Any irregularities in pain, touch, and motion sensations
   f. Cranial nerves
      (1) olfactory
      (2) optic
      (3) oculomotor
      (4) trochlear
      (5) trigeminal (motor and sensory)
      (6) abducens
      (7) facial
      (8) acoustic
      (9) glossopharyngeal
      (10) vagus
      (11) spinal accessory
      (12) hypoglossal
   g. Stereognosis
   h. Two-point discrimination
   i. Graphesthesia

PART 4

NORMAL FINDINGS OF THE ADULT PHYSICAL EXAMINATION BY ASSESSMENT PROCEDURE

AREA EXAMINED	ASSESSMENT	NORMAL FINDINGS
Assess vital functions	Temperature	98.6° F, 37° C
	Blood pressure	Upper limits 140/90
	Pulse	60 to 90/min, regular rhythm
	Height and weight	Refer to reference charts
	Vision test	
	Snellen	20/20 OU
	Near vision	20/20 OU
PATIENT IN SITTING POSITION		
Examine hands	Surface characteristics	Smooth, warm, intact
	Characteristics of nails	Smooth, hard, no thickening
	Clubbing	No clubbing noted
	Skeletal characteristics	No deformity, tenderness, or crepitations
	Range of motion (ROM)	Full ROM without pain
	Finger and hand strength	Bilaterally equal and firm grip

AREA EXAMINED	ASSESSMENT	NORMAL FINDINGS
Examine arms from hands to shoulders	Skin surface	Smooth, warm, intact
	Muscle strength	Bilaterally equal and strong
	ROM of all joints	Full ROM without pain
	Radial pulses	Bilaterally equal, regular, and strong
	Epitrochlear lymph nodes	Nodes not palpable
Examine head and neck	Facial characteristics and symmetry	Normocephalic, symmetrical
	Skin surface characteristics	Smooth, warm, intact without lesions
	Symmetry and external characteristics of eyes and ears	Eyes and ears symmetrical
		Eyebrows, lids, and lashes intact without deformity, ptosis, or lesions
		Conjunctiva, cornea, and sclera clear
		Ears have smooth auricles without lesions or discharge
	Hair characteristics	Evenly distributed, scalp without flaking, lesions, or tenderness
	Palpate facial bones and sinuses	Nontender
	Evaluate temporomandibular joint (TMJ), clench teeth (CN V)	Joint fully mobile, no tenderness or crepitus
	Clench eyes tightly, wrinkle forehead, stick tongue out, puff cheeks (CN VII, XII)	Performs all tasks easily, symmetrical responses
	Pupillary response; accommodation (CN II, III)	Pupils equal, round, react to light and accommodation (PERRLA)

Cover/uncover test	Eyes symmetrical without deviation of gaze
Extraocular eye movements: vision field testing (CN III, IV, VI)	Both eyes show coordination; parallel movement through the 6 cardinal fields of gaze
Internal eye exam: reflex, disc, cup vessels, retinal surface, vitreous, maculae	Red reflex present, disc is round, cream color, margin well defined, 2:3 A/V vessel ratio, vitreous is clear, retina red/orange, no exudates or lesions, maculae 2 DD from disc
Hearing evaluation (CN VIII)	Hears ticking watch or whisper at 2 feet (60 cm)
Otoscope exam of ear canal and tympanic membrane (TM)	External canal without lesions, some cerumen normal, TM intact, gray, landmarks visible
Rinne's test and Weber's test (CN VIII)	Rinne's: AC > BC Weber's: equal lateralization
Nose: structure, septum position, turbinates	Nose straight, nostrils patent, mucosa pink and moist
Evaluation of smell (CN I)	Odors properly identified
Mouth: gums, gingivobuccal fornices, buccal mucosa, palates	Lips moist and without lesions, mucosa, palates, and gingivae pink and without lesions
Teeth: number, color, characteristics	Thirty-two teeth present, firmly seated, and without caries or debris
Tongue: symmetry, movement, color, surface characteristics	Midline and symmetrical, pink, no lesions
Floor of mouth: color, surface characteristics	Pink, without lesions

AREA EXAMINED	ASSESSMENT	NORMAL FINDINGS
	Oropharynx: mouth odor, uvula, tonsils, posterior pharynx	Pink, no lesions, swelling, or exudate, uvula midline, tonsils present or absent, no foul odor present
	Gag reflex (CN IX, X)	Gag reflex present
	ROM of head and neck	Full and strong ROM without discomfort
	Push shoulders up against examiner's hands (CN XI)	Bilaterally strong and equal muscle response
	Carotid pulses	Symmetrical, strong, regular
	Jugular venous distention	Not present in sitting position
	Neck evaluation: thyroid, lymph nodes	Neck symmetrical, thyroid not palpable, lymph nodes not palpable
	Light sensation evaluation to forehead, cheeks, chin (CN V)	Feels the light sensation at all places touched
Assess posterior and lateral chest	Observe and palpate symmetry and muscle development, spine position, posture	Muscles bilaterally equal, appears appropriate for age, spine has normal shape with no deformities, slight kyphosis noted, AP chest diameter less than lateral chest diameter
	Observe respiration movement, quality of respirations	Diaphragmatic breathing, bilaterally equal excursion
	Palpate chest wall for fremitus	Tactile fremitus bilaterally equal
	Percuss for tone over chest wall	Resonant percussion tone throughout over lung fields

	Percuss CVA for tenderness	No CVA tenderness over kidneys
	Inspect, palpate, and percuss along lateral chest wall	Same as findings over posterior chest wall
	Auscultate chest walls for breath sounds	Vesicular breath sounds over most lung fields, bilaterally equal sounds throughout
Assess anterior chest	Inspect skin color, lesions, muscular and skeletal symmetry	Skin without lesions, adequate hydration, muscles bilaterally equal
	Observe chest wall movement during respiration	Chest wall moves bilaterally equally with respirations
	Observe ease of respirations	Breathing without difficulty, posturing, or splinting

Female Breasts

Size, symmetry, breast or nipple deviation	Breasts equal in size and position, no nipple deviation; areolar area intact and smooth, bilaterally equal pigmentation
Evaluate breast tissue during ROM of shoulders	Breasts appear smooth, without masses, bulges, retractions, or skin lesions, striae may be present

1. Arms extended over head
2. Hands behind head
3. Hands behind small of back
4. Hands pushed tightly against each other at shoulder level
5. Leans over so breasts fall away from chest wall

AREA EXAMINED	ASSESSMENT	NORMAL FINDINGS
	Male Breasts	
	Size, symmetry, nipple discharge, enlargement	Smooth skin without masses, retractions, bulges, or skin lesions
	All Patients	
	Palpate anterior chest wall for stability, muscle or skeletal tenderness, or crepitations	Chest wall firm, without bulging, retractions, or asymmetry
	Palpate precordium for thrills, heaves, pulsations	No thrills or heaves palpated, slight pulsation felt over chest wall
	Locate PMI	PMI palpable at the 5th ICS, approximately 8 cm from the midsternal line
	Palpate fremitus	Tactile fremitus bilaterally equal
	Percuss anterior chest for resonance	Resonant tone percussed over most lung fields
	Palpate all breast quadrants and areolae for lumps	Breasts firm, smooth texture throughout, without masses, bulges, retractions, or tenderness
	Palpate nipples for tissue characteristics and discharge	Nipples erect, no discharge, not tender to palpation
	Palpate lymph node areas associated with lymphatic drainage of breasts	No lymph nodes palpable

| | Auscultate breath sounds of anterior chest for rate, quality, type, and presence of adventitious sounds | Vesicular breath sounds over most lung fields, bilaterally equal sounds throughout |
| | Auscultate heart (diaphragm and bell) over aortic, pulmonary, Erb's point, tricuspid, and apical areas; note rate, rhythm, location, intensity, timing, frequency, splitting, and murmurs | Rate = 60 to 90/min, regular rhythm, S1, S2 heard in all locations, S1 louder at apex and longer in duration, S2 louder at base and shorter in duration (splitting may be normally heard in young persons over pulmonary area), no extra sounds or murmurs |

PATIENT IN LYING DOWN OR FOWLER'S POSITION

Assess anterior chest	Inspect JVP for height seen above sternal angle	JVP at level of sternal angle when patient is elevated to 30 degrees
	Repeat breast inspection while patient is in recumbent position	Same as previously described
	Repeat breast palpation while patient is in recumbent position	Same as previously described
	Repeat palpation of anterior chest wall for cardiac movement, thrills, heaves, or pulsations	Same as previously described
	Repeat auscultation of the five areas over the heart (use diaphragm and bell)	Same as previously described
	Turn patient to the left side and repeat cardiac auscultation	Same as previously described

AREA EXAMINED	ASSESSMENT	NORMAL FINDINGS
Assess abdomen from epigastric region to pubis	Observe skin characteristics from pubis to epigastrium for scars, lesions, vascularity, bulges, and position and characteristics of the navel	Skin smooth, warm, well hydrated, and intact, no lesions, scars, rashes, discolorations, inflammation, or bulges, umbilicus centered, no visible hernia or ulceration
	Observe abdominal contour	Contour rounded and symmetrical
	Observe movement of abdomen, peristalsis, and pulsations	No peristalsis noted (slight pulsations may be seen above umbilicus and over aorta in thin individuals)
	Auscultate all quadrants of abdomen for bowel sounds, bruits, and venous hum	Bowel sounds (gurgles and clicks) present in all 4 quadrants: 5 to 30/min, no bruits or venous hums heard
	Percuss all quadrants and epigastric region of abdomen for tone	Tympanic sounds heard in all quadrants, dullness may be heard over superpubic region
	Percuss upper and lower liver borders for position and tenderness	Lower border of liver percussed at costal margin or slightly below. Upper border percussed between 5th and 7th ICS, midclavicular liver span is 6 to 12 cm, midsternal liver span is 4 to 8 cm, percussion tone over liver is dull, liver nontender to percussion
	Percuss left midaxillary line for splenic dullness	Area of splenic dullness extends from 6th to 10th ribs

Light palpation of all four quadrants for tenderness, guarding, and masses	Abdomen relaxed and smooth, no tenderness or masses felt
Deep palpation of all four quadrants for tenderness, guarding, and masses	May exhibit some tenderness over midline at xiphoid, over cecum, and over sigmoid colon, aorta may be palpated at epigastrium, feces may be palpated along descending colon, no masses palpated
Deep palpation of right costal margin for liver border	Liver often not palpable, may "bump" downward against fingers, liver border should be smooth and nontender
Deep palpation of left costal margin for splenic border	Spleen not normally palpable
Deep palpation of abdomen for right and left kidneys	Contour should be smooth and nontender (lower poles of kidneys may be felt in a thin individual)
Evaluate abdominal reflexes with pointed instrument (evaluation of T8 through T12)	Abdominal muscles contract slightly, bilaterally equal response, umbilicus moves slightly toward area of stimulus
Client raises head for evaluation of flexion and strength of abdominal muscles	ROM of neck permits chin to chest flexion, abdominal muscles firm, prominent, and permit patient to raise head easily off exam table
Light palpation of inguinal region for lymph nodes, femoral pulses, and bulges	Nodes not palpable, strong bilaterally equal femoral pulses palpated, inguinal region without bulges or tenderness

55

AREA EXAMINED	ASSESSMENT	NORMAL FINDINGS
Assess lower limbs and hips	Assess feet and legs for skin integrity, vascular sufficiency, pulses, and skeletal formation of legs, feet, and toes	Skin intact without lesions or dryness, limbs appear well hydrated without evidence of pallor, venous stasis, or edema, bilaterally equal and strong pulses at popliteal, dorsalis pedis, and posterior tibial positions, feet and toes without swelling or deformity, toes and feet maintain extended and straight positions
	Palpate feet and lower legs for temperature, tenderness, and deformities	Legs and feet warm to touch, good capillary refill following blanching technique, no tenderness with palpation
	Perform ROM and muscle strength of hips, knees, ankles, feet, and toes	Full active ROM of all joints without limitations or discomfort
	Palpate hips for stability	Hips bilaterally symmetrical and stable, no discomfort with palpation
Assess genital, pelvic region, and rectum	*Men*	
	Inspect and palpate external genitalia, including pubic hair, penis, scrotum, testes, epididymides, and vas deferens (move patient to lateral knee chest position)	Pubic hair has triangular configuration with hair extending up linea alba to umbilicus, penis without lesions, induration, or discharge, scrotal contents palpated without tenderness or masses
	Inspect perianal area and anus for surface characteristics	Perianal and anal surfaces show no presence of rashes, inflammation, masses, or hemorrhoids

Palpate anus, rectum, and prostate with gloved finger, note stool characteristics when gloved finger is removed	Good sphincter tone, anal and rectal mucosa smooth and without masses, palpated prostate bilobed and firm without tenderness or enlargement, stool noted as brown and soft

Women

Position patient in lithotomy position	
Inspect and palpate external genitalia, including pubic hair, labia, clitoris, urethral and vaginal orifices, perineal and perianal area, and anus	Hair distribution inverted triangular shape, no masses or lesions noted, labia, vestibule, and urethra intact without redness or tenderness, no foul odor or discharge noted, perineum intact
Insert speculum and inspect surface characteristics of vagina and cervix	Cervix midline, pink, firm, and mobile without lesions, round or slit shape, vaginal surface rugous and moist
Remove speculum and perform bimanual palpation of vagina, cervix, uterus, and adnexa to assess form, size, and characteristics	Uterus pear shaped 5 to 8 cm long, fundus firm and anterior, contour smooth and nontender, freely moveable with palpation, ovaries and tubes may not be palpable, no masses or tenderness palpated
Perform vaginal-rectal examination to assess recto-vaginal septum and pouch, surface characteristics, and broad ligament	Septum smooth and firm, cul-de-sac and rectum without nodules, tenderness, or masses
Perform rectal exam with gloved finger to assess anal sphincter tone and surface characteristics, note stool characteristics when gloved finger is removed	Good sphincter tone, anal and rectal mucosa smooth and without masses, stool noted as brown and soft

AREA EXAMINED	ASSESSMENT	NORMAL FINDINGS
PATIENT IN SITTING POSITION		
Assess neurological system	Observe patient moving from lying to sitting position, note use of muscles, ease of movement, and coordination	Good muscle coordination and strength, pushes off with arms and hands, balance OK, no noted limitations or weaknesses
	Test sensory function of neurological system by using sharp and dull, deep and light sensation of forehead, paranasal sinus areas, hands, lower arms, feet, and lower legs	Sensations correctly interpreted as sharp or dull, and light or deep, at all areas tested
	Bilaterally test and compare vibratory sensation of bony areas of ankle, wrist, and sternum	Sense of vibration equally felt at all positions tested
	Test 2-point discrimination of back of hand, thigh, and back	Can distinguish 2-point discrimination Hands: 8 to 12 mm Thigh: 60 to 75 mm Back: 40 to 70 mm
	Test stereognosis or graphesthesia	Appropriate identification of object or written number
	Test fine motor proprioception and cerebellar function and coordination of upper extremities by instinct, patient to do at least 2 of the following: 1. Alternating pronation and supination of forearms	Purposeful and bilaterally equal response to all commands, movements done quickly and with precision

2. Touching nose with alternating index fingers
3. Rapidly alternating finger movements to thumb
4. Rapid movement of index finger between nose and examiner's finger

Test and bilaterally compare fine motor function and coordination of lower extremities by instructing patient to run heel down tibia of opposite leg	Purposeful and bilaterally equal response, movements done quickly and with precision
Alternately crossing legs over knee	Purposeful and bilaterally equal response
Test and bilaterally compare deep tendon reflexes including biceps, triceps, brachioradialis, patellar, and Achilles tendons	Deep tendon reflexes (DTR) intact, bilaterally equal, quick, brisk response

PATIENT IN STANDING POSITION

Male scrotum and hernia evaluation	Palpate scrotum and inguinal regions for characteristics and hernia	Scrotum palpated without tenderness or masses, all contents freely moveable and smooth, no bulges felt with hernia evaluation (triangular slit opening of inguinal ring may or may not admit examiner's finger)
Assess neurological and musculo-skeletal system	Assess gait	Gait smooth, coordinated, rhythmic, walks with ease, arms extended to sides, stands erect

AREA EXAMINED	ASSESSMENT	NORMAL FINDINGS
	Observe and palpate spine as patient stands and bends forward to touch toes	Spine straight, iliac crests of equal heights, shoulders of equal heights, convexity of thoracic spine noted
	Stabilize patient at waist and evaluate hyper-extension, lateral bending, and rotation of upper trunk	ROM with ease in all directions, no discomfort or dizziness
	Assess proprioception and cerebellar and motor function by using at least 2 of the following: 1. Romberg's test (eyes closed) 2. Walk straight, heel-toe formation 3. Stand on one foot and then the other (eyes closed) 4. Hop in place on one foot and then the other 5. Perform knee bends	Able to follow directions during all techniques, maintains upright posture with no assistance, balance maintained throughout

NERVE	METHOD TO TEST	NORMAL RESULTS
I. Olfactory nerve	Eyes closed: patient smells an aromatic substance	Patient correctly identifies odor
II. Optic nerve	Measure distant vision using a Snellen eye chart	20/20 OU
III. Oculomotor nerve IV. Trochlear nerve VI. Abducens nerve	Measure six cardinal fields of gaze	Moves eyes in all six fields of gaze

Six cardinal fields of gaze

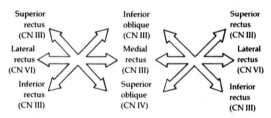

V. Trigeminal nerve	Measure motor component: instruct patient to clench teeth	Bilaterally strong muscle contraction
	Measure sensory component: lightly touch forehead with a cotton wisp	Tickle sensation equally present over palpated areas

Evaluation of Cranial Nerves—cont'd

NERVE	METHOD TO TEST	NORMAL RESULTS
	Deep sensation: use alternating sharp and blunt palpation over forehead and sinus area	Differentiates between sharp and dull sensations
	Corneal reflex: lightly touch cornea with a cotton wisp	Bilaterally blinks to corneal touch
VII. Facial nerve	Inspect face at rest and during conversation	Symmetrical face
	Instruct patient to raise eyebrows, frown, close eyes tightly, show teeth, smile, and puff out cheeks	Symmetrical face
	Evaluate taste on tongue (anterior ⅔ of tongue)	Correctly identifies taste
VIII. Acoustic nerve	Assess vestibular function: use Romberg's test (have patient stand with feet together and eyes closed, watch for steadiness of stance)	Maintains body position
	Whispered voice, ticking watch	Bilaterally equal sounds
	Rinne's test	AC > BC
	Weber's test	Bilaterally equal sounds
IX. Glossopharyngeal nerve	Instruct patient to say "ah"	Bilaterally equal upward movement of soft palate and uvula
X. Vagus nerve	Evaluate taste on posterior ⅓ of tongue	Correctly identifies taste
	Evaluate gag reflex	Gag initiated

XI. Spinal accessory nerve	Have patient shrug shoulders against examiner's hands	Strong and symmetrical movements
	Have patient turn head side to side against examiner's hands	Strong and symmetrical movements
XII. Hypoglossal nerve	Evaluate motor movement of tongue	Full movement of tongue

GLASGOW COMA SCALE*

Best eye opening response		
(Record "C" if eyes closed by swelling)	Spontaneously	4
	To speech	3
	To pain	2
	No response	1
Best motor response to painful stimuli		
(Record best upper limb response)	Obeys verbal command	6
	Localizes pain	5
	Flexion—withdrawal	4
	Flexion—abnormal†	3
	Extension—abnormal‡	2
	No response	1
Best verbal response		
(Record "E" if endotracheal tube in place, "T" is tracheostomy tube in place)	Oriented X 3	5
	Conversation confused	4
	Speech inappropriate	3
	Sounds incomprehensible	2
	No response	1

NOTE: The Glasgow Coma Scale also correlates well with survival and cognitive outcome. Patients with low scores (3, 4) have a high mortality and poor prognosis for cognitive recovery, whereas patients with high scores (greater than 8) have a good prognosis for recovery.

*Eye + Motor + Verbal = 3 to 15
†Abnormal flexion—decorticate
‡Abnormal extension—decerebrate

PART 5

EXAMINATION OF THE CHILD

AGE AND PREPARATION	PROCEDURES
1. Newborn to 6 months: undressed, lying on examination table	1. Obtain history, highlighting developmental or problem areas
	2. Check vital signs: temperature, pulse, respiration
	3. Record weight, length, chest and head circumference
	4. Observe child lying on examination table: note color, general health, body symmetry, gross motor movement, alertness, gross and fine motor development, language development, social adaptive development, skin characteristics, and response to sound and visual stimulation
	5. Examine and manipulate hands, arms, shoulders, feet, legs, note ROM and tone
	6. Examine skin over extremities, chest, abdomen, and back
	7. Auscultate thorax, lungs, heart, abdomen
	8. Palpate and examine external characteristics of head, neck, face, axillary region
	9. Palpate thorax, abdomen, and umbilical area

AGE AND PREPARATION	PROCEDURES
	10. Observe and palpate external genitalia, inguinal area, and hip stability
	11. Examine eyes with ophthalmoscope
	12. Examine mouth, teeth (development), tongue, posterior pharynx, nose
	13. Examine ears with otoscope
2. Six months to 2 years: child in diaper, sitting on parent's lap; examiner's chair should be in front of parent's chair and examiner's knees should touch parent's; during supine examination, child may lie on parent's and examiner's laps	1. Obtain history, highlighting developmental or problem areas
	2. Perform developmental, social, vision, speech, hearing, and fine and gross motor assessment during play and initial "get acquainted" period
	3. Record weight, length, and chest and head circumference (until 18 months)
	4. Check vital signs, including blood pressure in children over 18 months of age, may be postponed until later if child becomes agitated
	5. Auscultate lungs and heart
	6. Examine skin over extremities, chest, abdomen, and back
	7. Examine and manipulate hands, arms, shoulders, feet, legs, note ROM and tone
	8. Palpate and examine external characteristics of head, neck, face, axillary region
	9. Auscultate abdomen with child in supine position on parent's and examiner's laps
	10. Palpate thorax, abdomen, and umbilical area

11. Observe and palpate external genitalia, inguinal area, and hip stability
12. Examine eyes with ophthalmoscope
13. Examine mouth, teeth (development), tongue, posterior pharynx, nose
14. Examine ears with otoscope

3. Two to 4 years: undressed to underpants, may be examined either on parent's lap or on examination table, much of assessment may be informal as examiner observes and plays with child

Same as for child from 6 months to 2 years

4. Four to 6 years: undressed to underpants, sitting on examination table, assessment should move toward adult format, child's developmental immaturity may necessitate that examiner alter various examination techniques to facilitate child's participation and correct response

Same as for child from 6 months to 2 years

5. Over 6 years old: in gown on examination table

Same as for adult patient

Normal Developmental Guidelines for the Child

AGE	FINE MOTOR	GROSS MOTOR	SOCIAL/ ADAPTIVE	LANGUAGE
1 month	Follows with eyes to midline	Turns head to side, keeps knees tucked under abdomen, gross head lag and rounded swayed back (when pulled to sitting position)	Regards face	Responds to bell
2 months	Follows objects well, may not follow past midline (major developmental milestone)	Holds head in same plane as rest of body, can raise head and maintain position, looks downward	Smiles responsively	Vocalizes (not crying)
3 months	Follows past midline, puts hands together (when in supine position), will hold hands in front of face	Raises head to 45-degree angle, maintains posture, looks around with head, may turn from prone to side position, shows only slight head lag (when pulled to sitting position)		Laughs
4 months	Grasps rattle, plays with hands together	Actively lifts head up and looks around, will roll from prone to supine position, no longer has head lag (when pulled to sitting		Squeals

		position), attempts to maintain some weight support (when held in standing position)		
5 months	Can reach and pick up object, may play with toes	Pushes up from prone position and maintains weight on forearms, rolls from prone to supine and back to prone, maintains straight back (when in sitting position)	Smiles spontaneously	
6 months	Holds spoon or rattle, drops object and reaches for second offered object	Begins to raise abdomen off table, sits (posture still shaky), may sit with legs apart, holds arms straight as prop between legs, supports almost full weight (when pulled to standing position)		
7 months	Transfers object 1 hand to other, grasps objects in each hand	Sits alone, still uses hands for support, bounces (when held in standing position), puts feet to mouth		
8 months	Beginning thumb-finger grasping	Sits securely without support (major developmental milestone)	Feeds self crackers	Turns to voice

Data from Frankenburg, W.K., Sciarillo, W., and Burgess, D.: J. Pediatr. 99(6):995-999, 1981.

Normal Developmental Guidelines for the Child—cont'd

AGE	FINE MOTOR	GROSS MOTOR	SOCIAL/ ADAPTIVE	LANGUAGE
9 months	Continued development of thumb-finger grasp, may bang objects together	Steady sitting, can lean forward and still maintain position, begins creeping (abdomen off floor), stands holding onto stabilizing object (when placed in that position), still may not be able to pull self into standing position		
10 months	Practices picking up small objects, points with 1 finger, offers toys to people but unable to let go of objects	Can pull self into standing position, unable to let self down again	Plays peek-a-boo	
11 months		Moves about room holding onto objects, preparing to walk independently, wide-base stance, stands securely (holding on with one hand)		Imitates speech sound
12 months (1 year)	Holds cup and spoon and feeds self fairly well (with practice), offers toys and releases them	Able to twist and turn and maintain posture, sits from standing position, stands alone at least momentarily		"Dada" or "mama" specific

14 months		Plays pat-a-cake		
15 months	Puts raisins into bottle, takes off shoes, and pulls toys	Walks alone well, seats self in chair		
16 months		Plays ball with examiner		
18 months	Holds crayon, scribbles spontaneously (major developmental milestone)	Walks up and down stairs holding hand, shows running ability		
20 months		Imitates housework		Three words other than "mama" or "dada"
24 months (2 years)	Turns doorknob, takes off shoes and socks, builds 2-block tower, dumps raisins from bottle (following demonstration)	Walks up stairs by self (2 feet on each step), walks backward, kicks ball	Uses spoon	
28 months				Combines 2 words
30 months (2½ years)	Builds 4-block tower, scribbling techniques continue, feeds self with increased neatness, dumps raisins from bottle spontaneously	Jumps from object, walking becomes more stable, wide-base gait decreases, throws ball overhanded		

Normal Developmental Guidelines for the Child—cont'd

AGE	FINE MOTOR	GROSS MOTOR	SOCIAL/ ADAPTIVE	LANGUAGE
36 months (3 years)	Unbuttons front buttons, copies vertical lines within 30 degrees, copies ○, builds 8-cube tower	Walks up stairs (alternating feet on steps), walks down stairs (2 feet on each step), pedals tricycle, jumps in place, performs broad jump	Pulls on shoes	Follows 2 or 3 simple directions
48 months (4 years)	Copies +, picks longer line (3 out of 3 times)	Walks down stairs (alternating feet on steps), buttons large front buttons, balances on 1 foot for approximately 5 seconds	Dresses with supervision	Gives first and last names
60 months (5 years)	Dresses self with minimal assistance, draws 3-part human figure, draws □ (following demonstration), colors within lines	Hops on 1 foot, catches ball bounced to child (2 out of 3 times), demonstrates heel-toe walking	Dresses without supervision	Recognizes 3 colors

PART 6

HISTORY AND PHYSICAL EXAMINATION REPORT

DOCUMENTATION FORMAT

1. **Subjective data base**
   a. Biographical data
   b. Reason for visit
   c. Present health status
   d. Current health data: medications, allergies, immunizations, last exam
   e. Past health status: childhood illnesses, serious or chronic illnesses, serious accidents or injuries, hospitalizations, operations, emotional health, obstetrical health
   f. Family history
   g. Review of physiological systems: general, nutritional, integumentary, head, eyes, ears, nose, mouth, neck, breast, cardiovascular, respiratory, hematolymphatic, gastrointestinal, urinary, genital, musculoskeletal, central nervous system, endocrine, and allergic and immunological
   h. Psychological history: general status, response to illness
   i. Social history: significant others, occupational history, educational level, ADL, habits, financial status
   j. Health maintenance efforts: maintenance of self-health, health care patterns
   k. Environmental health: general assessment, employment, home, neighborhood, community

2. **Physical assessment**
   a. Vital statistics: height, weight, temperature, pulse, blood pressure (both arms, lying, sitting, standing)
   b. General statement of appearance
   c. Mental health
   d. Integumentary: skin, nails, body hair
   e. Head and neck: scalp, hair, face, neck, lymph nodes, thyroid, trachea, sinuses
   f. Nose: patency, surface characteristics
   g. Mouth, pharynx: oral cavity characteristics, teeth, tongue, voice, tonsillar area, and posterior pharynx

h. Ear and auditory: external ear, canal, TM characteristics, hearing, Rinne's and Weber's tests
i. Eye and visual: external eye characteristics, vision, eye movement, ophthalmoscopy
j. Thorax and lungs: thorax characteristics, breathing pattern and rate, percussion tone, auscultatory characteristics
k. Cardiovascular: all pulses, blood pressure, extremity circulation, precordium characteristics, heart sounds
l. Breast: surface characteristics, areolae and nipples, palpation characteristics, lymphatic assessment, breast self-examination assessment
m. Abdominal, rectal: contour, surface characteristics, bowel sounds, percussion tones, palpation characteristics, liver and spleen, bladder, kidney characteristics, CVA tenderness, hernias, rectal examination findings
n. Genital
   (1) Women: external genitalia characteristics, internal (cervix, vagina, uterus), adnexa characteristics
   (2) Men: external genitalia characteristics, palpation characteristics of penis and scrotum, inguinal hernia evaluation
o. Musculoskeletal: muscular development and strength, skeletal and joint characteristics and symmetry, range of motion
p. Neurological: orientation, intactness of CN I to XII, coordination of fine and gross motor movements and gait, sensory evaluation, reflexes

3. **Risk profile**: items from the patient's history and physical assessment that might indicate risk to the overall health state (the data base in Part I details these potential problems)

4. **Problem list**: a synthesis of those items currently identified as stresses for the patient (may be physiological, sociological, psychological, or a combination of these). The problems are those items that reduce the patient's overall level of health. Once the problems are listed and assigned a priority, the examiner can then decide which are within his or her scope of practice to handle and which must be referred.

PART 7

REFERENCE DATA

ABBREVIATIONS

A&P anterior and posterior, auscultation and percussion

A&W alive and well

abd abdomen, abdominal

AJ ankle jerk

AK above knee

ANS autonomic nervous system

BK below knee

BS bowel sounds, breath sounds

CC chief complaint

CHD childhood disease, congenital heart disease, coronary heart disease

CHF congestive heart failure

CNS central nervous system

COPD chronic obstructive pulmonary disease

CV cardiovascular

CVA costovertebral angle, cerebrovascular accident

CVP central venous pressure

Cx cervix

D&C dilatation and curettage

DM diabetes mellitus

DOB date of birth

DTR deep tendon reflex

Dx diagnosis

ECG, EKG electrocardiogram, electrocardiograph

EENT eye, ear, nose, and throat

ENT ear, nose, and throat

EOM extraocular movement

FB foreign body

FH family history

Fx fracture

GB gallbladder

GU genitourinary

GYN gynecological

HOPI history of present illness
Hx history

ICS intercostal space
IOP intraocular pressure

JVP jugular venous pressure

lat lateral
LCM left costal margin
LLQ left lower quadrant (abdomen)
LMP last menstrual period
LS lumbosacral
LSB left sternal border
LUL left upper lobe (lung)
LUQ left upper quadrant (abdomen)

MSL midsternal line

N&T nose and throat
N&V nausea and vomiting
NSR normal sinus rhythm

OD right eye
OM otitis media
OS left eye
OU both eyes

P&A percussion and auscultation
PE physical examination
PERRLA pupils equal, round, react to light and accommodation
PI present illness
PID pelvic inflammatory disease
PMH past medical history
PMI point of maximum impulse, point of maximum intensity
PVC premature ventricular contraction

RCM right costal margin
REM rapid eye movement
RLQ right lower quadrant (abdomen)
ROM range of motion
RUQ right upper quadrant (abdomen)

SQ subcutaneous

T&A tonsillectomy and adenoidectomy
TM tympanic membrane
TMJ temporomandibular joint
TPR temperature, pulse, and respiration

URI upper respiratory infection
UTI urinary tract infection

CONVERSION TABLES

Length

INCH	CM	CM	INCH
1	2.5	1	0.4
2	5.1	2	0.8
4	10.2	3	1.2
6	15.2	4	1.6
8	20.3	5	2.0
10	25.4	6	2.4
20	50.8	8	3.1
30	76.2	10	3.9
40	101.6	20	7.9
50	127.0	30	11.8
60	152.4	40	15.7
70	177.8	50	19.7
80	203.2	60	23.6
90	227.6	70	27.6
100	254.0	80	31.5
150	381.0	90	35.4
200	508.0	100	39.4

1 inch =
2.54 cm

1 cm =
0.3937 inch

Weight

LB	KG	KG	LB
1	0.5	1	2.2
2	0.9	2	4.4
4	1.8	3	6.6
6	2.7	4	8.8
8	3.6	5	11.0
10	4.5	6	13.2
20	9.1	8	17.6
30	13.6	10	22
40	18.2	20	44
50	22.7	30	66
60	27.3	40	88
70	31.8	50	110
80	36.4	60	132
90	40.9	70	154
100	45.4	80	176
150	66.2	90	198
200	90.8	100	220

1 lb =
0.454 kg

1 kg =
2.204 lb

HEIGHT AND WEIGHT TABLES FOR ADULTS

Desirable Weights for Men
(According to Frame, Ages 25-59)

HEIGHT*		WEIGHT†		
FEET	INCHES	SMALL FRAME	MEDIUM FRAME	LARGE FRAME
5	2	128-134	131-141	138-150
5	3	130-136	133-143	140-153
5	4	132-138	135-145	142-156
5	5	134-140	137-148	144-160
5	6	136-142	139-151	146-164
5	7	138-145	142-154	149-168
5	8	140-148	145-157	152-172
5	9	142-151	148-160	155-176
5	10	144-154	151-163	158-180
5	11	146-157	154-166	161-184
6	0	149-160	157-170	164-188
6	1	152-164	160-174	168-192
6	2	155-168	164-178	172-197
6	3	158-172	167-182	176-202
6	4	162-176	171-187	181-207

Data from: Build study, 1979, Society of Actuaries and Association of Life Insurance Medical Directors of America, 1980. Copyright 1983 Metropolitan Life Insurance Company.
*Shoes with 1-inch heels.
†Weight in pounds (in indoor clothing weighing 5 pounds).

Desirable Weights for Women
(According to Frame, Ages 25-59)

HEIGHT*		WEIGHT†		
FEET	INCHES	SMALL FRAME	MEDIUM FRAME	LARGE FRAME
4	10	102-111	109-121	118-131
4	11	103-113	111-123	120-134
5	0	104-114	113-126	122-137
5	1	106-118	115-129	125-140
5	2	108-121	118-132	128-143
5	3	111-123	121-135	131-147
5	4	114-127	124-138	134-151
5	5	117-130	127-141	137-155
5	6	120-133	130-144	140-159
5	7	123-136	133-147	143-163
5	8	126-139	136-150	146-167
5	9	129-142	139-153	149-170
5	10	132-145	142-156	152-173
5	11	135-148	145-159	155-176
6	0	138-151	148-162	158-179

Data from: Build study, 1979, Society of Actuaries and Association of Life Insurance Medical Directors of America, 1980. Copyright 1983 Metropolitan Life Insurance Company.
*Shoes with 1-inch heels.
†Weight in pounds (in indoor clothing weighing 5 pounds).

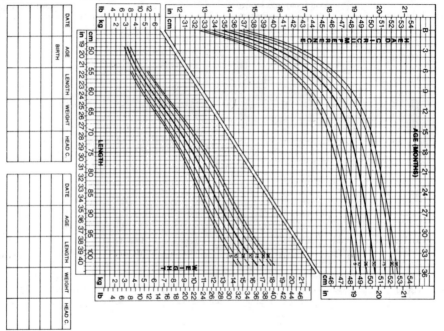

DATE	AGE	LENGTH	WEIGHT	HEAD C.
	BIRTH			

DATE	AGE	LENGTH	WEIGHT	HEAD C.

(Adapted from Hamill, P.V.V., and others: Physical growth: National Center for Health Statistics percentiles, Am. J. Clin. Nutr. 32:607–629, 1979. Data from the Fels Research Institute, Wright State University School of Medicine, Yellow Springs, Ohio. Provided as a service of Ross Laboratories, 1980.)

GIRLS: BIRTH TO 36 MONTHS—PHYSICAL GROWTH, NCHS PERCENTILES

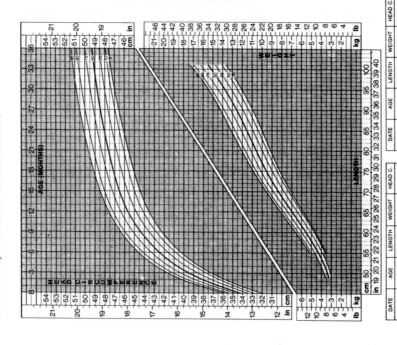

(Adapted from Hamill, P.V.V., and others: Physical growth: National Center for Health Statistics percentiles, Am. J. Clin. Nutr. 32:607-629, 1979. Data from the Fels Research Institute, Wright State University School of Medicine, Yellow Springs, Ohio. Provided as a service of Ross Laboratories, 1980.)

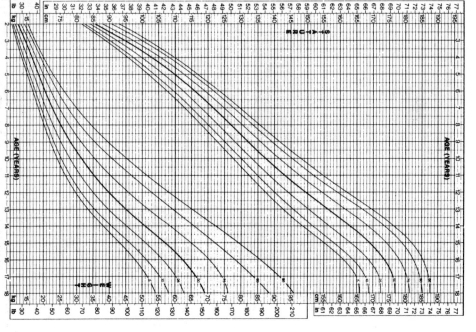

(Adapted from Hamill, P.V.V., and others: Physical growth: National Center for
Health Statistics percentiles, Am. J. Clin. Nutr. 32:607–629, 1979. Data from the
National Center for Health Statistics [NCHS], Hyattsville, Md. Provided as a service
of Ross Laboratories, 1980.)

GIRLS: 2 TO 18 YEARS—PHYSICAL GROWTH, NCHS PERCENTILES

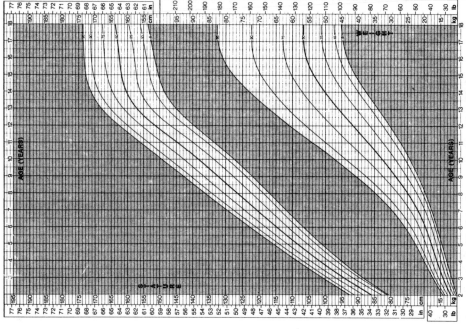

(Adapted from Hamill, P.V.V., and others: Physical growth: National Center for Health Statistics percentiles, Am. J. Clin. Nutr. 32:607-629, 1979. Data from the National Center for Health Statistics [NCHS], Hyattsville, Md. Provided as a service of Ross Laboratories, 1980.)

INCHES 1 2 3 4 5

95

874

2843

638 EWE XOO

8745 ЭШ OXO

6392 5 ШЕЭ OXO

428365 ШЕЭ XOX

374258 EШE OXO

937826 ШЕШ XOO

* 2 8 7 3 9 ШEШ ° ° °

	Point	Jaeger	distance equivalent
	26 16		$\frac{20}{200}$
			$\frac{20}{400}$
			$\frac{20}{800}$

Card is held in good light 14 inches from eye. Record vision for each eye separately with and without glasses. Presbyopic patients should read thru bifocal segment. Check myopes with glasses only.

METRIC 1 2 3 4 5 6 7 8 9 10 11 12 13 14

NOTES

NOTES

NOTES